VEGAN KIDNEY-FRIENDLY RECIPES

Delicious and Nutritious Meals to Support Kidney Health

Dr Lily Morgan

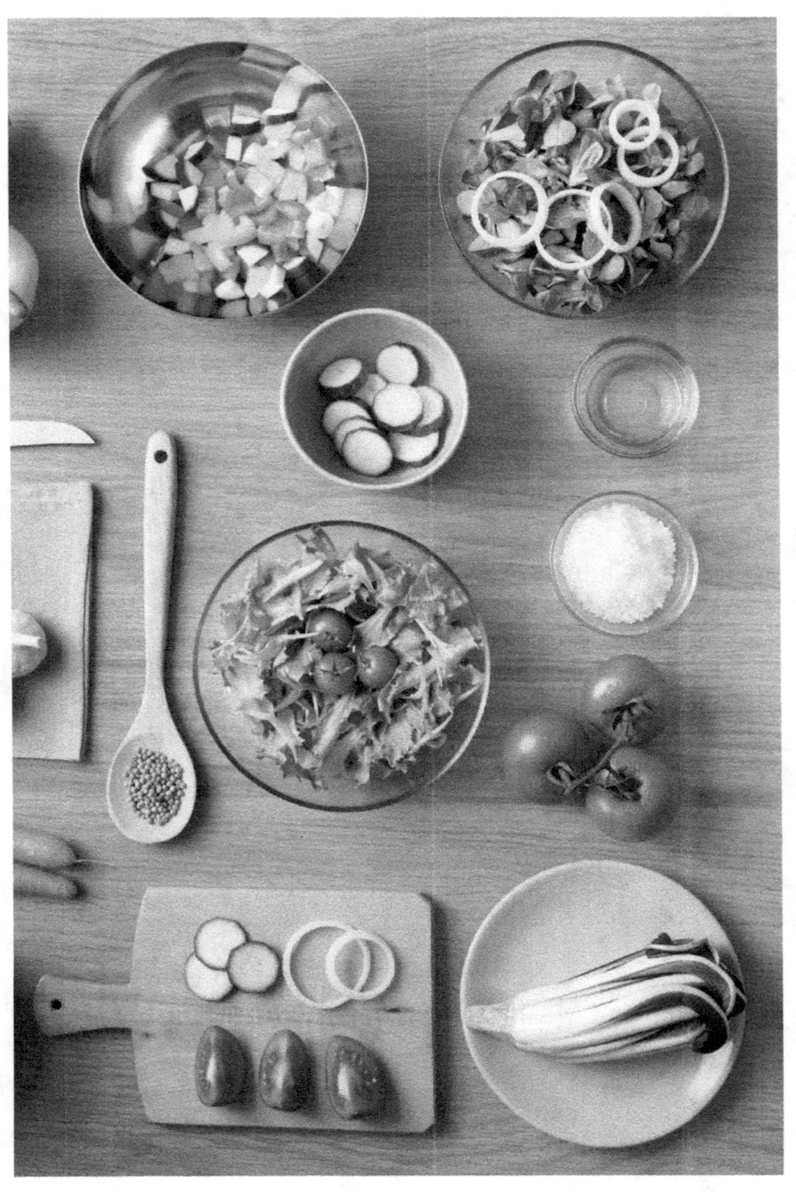

TABLE OF CONTENTS

INTRODUCTION 9

Chapter 1: 30-Day Meal Plan 12

Week 1 12

Week 2 14

Week 3 16

Week 4 18

Chapter 2: Breakfast Recipes...................... 23

Creamy Oatmeal with Berries................................ 23

Vegan Scrambled Tofu 24

Sweet Potato and Spinach Breakfast Burrito 25

Blueberry Banana Pancakes................................... 25

Chia Seed Pudding... 26

Avocado Toast with Tomato Salsa 27

Vegan Breakfast Smoothie 27

Quinoa and Fruit Bowl.. 28

Nutty Granola with Almond Milk............................ 28

Spinach and Mushroom Breakfast Quesadilla.............. 29

Zucchini and Tomato Frittata................................. 30

Cinnamon Raisin French Toast............................... 30

Vegan Breakfast Tacos 31

Peanut Butter and Banana Toast 32

Kidney-Friendly Green Smoothie.................................... 32

Chickpea Breakfast Hash 33

Vegan Chocolate Porridge 33

Mediterranean Breakfast Bowl 34

Chapter 3: Lunch Recipes.................................. 35

Kidney Bean and Quinoa Salad 35

Vegan Lentil Soup 36

Spaghetti with Vegan Bolognese 37

Black Bean and Corn Salad 38

Vegan Falafel Wraps... 39

Sweet Potato and Kale Salad 40

Vegan Minestrone Soup... 41

Spinach and Chickpea Salad... 42

Vegan Thai Peanut Noodles.. 43

Roasted Red Pepper Hummus Wrap................................ 44

Vegan Sushi Bowl.. 45

Vegan Butternut Squash Soup 45

Vegan Chickpea Curry.. 46

Vegan Stuffed Bell Peppers 47

Quinoa and Avocado Salad... 48

Vegan Caesar Salad 49

Vegan Lentil Tacos 50

Vegan Portobello Mushroom Burger................................ 51

Chapter 4: Dinner Recipes 52

Vegan Eggplant Parmesan 52

Kidney Bean Stew... 53

Vegan Tofu Stir-Fry.. 54

Vegan Spaghetti Aglio e Olio 55

Vegan Sweet Potato and Black Bean Chili.................... 56

Vegan Mushroom Risotto.. 57

Vegan Stuffed Acorn Squash... 58

Vegan Teriyaki Tempeh 59

Vegan Cauliflower Curry... 59

Vegan Spinach and Artichoke Pasta 60

Vegan Ratatouille.. 61

Vegan Lentil Loaf 62

Vegan Cilantro Lime Rice with Black Beans 63

Vegan Portobello Steak.. 64

Vegan Chickpea and Spinach Curry 65

Vegan Quinoa Stuffed Peppers... 65

Vegan Thai Green Curry.. 66

Vegan Asparagus and Lemon Risotto............................... 67

Chapter 5: Snacks and Appetizers 69

Vegan Guacamole... 69

Vegan Stuffed Mushrooms 70

Vegan Cucumber Rolls.. 71

Vegan Sweet Potato Fries 72

Vegan Salsa and Tortilla Chips.. 73

Vegan Edamame 74

Vegan Greek Salad Skewers 75

Vegan Roasted Red Pepper Dip...................................... 75

Vegan Avocado Bruschetta.. 76

Vegan Spinach and Artichoke Dip 77

Vegan Hummus and Veggie Sticks 78

Vegan Fruit Salad 79

Vegan Olive Tapenade.. 79

Vegan Roasted Chickpeas... 80

Vegan Stuffed Grape Leaves 81

Vegan Zucchini Chips... 82

Vegan Mini Caprese Skewers 82

Vegan Mixed Nuts 83

Chapter 6: Desserts 84

Vegan Banana Ice Cream.. 84

Vegan Chocolate Avocado Mousse 85

Vegan Berry Parfait 85

Vegan Baked Apples... 86

Vegan Coconut Rice Pudding... 87

Vegan Pumpkin Pie.. 87

Vegan Chia Seed Chocolate Pudding 88

Vegan Mixed Berry Crisp... 89

Vegan Chocolate Chip Cookies 89

Vegan Rice Krispie Treats 90

Vegan Lemon Sorbet 91

Vegan Strawberry Shortcake 91

Vegan Blueberry Cobbler 92

Vegan Chocolate Covered Strawberries 92

Vegan Almond and Coconut Energy Balls 93

Vegan Mango Sorbet 94

Vegan Watermelon Popsicles 94

Vegan Cinnamon Baked Pears.. 95

CONCLUSION 96

INTRODUCTION

Kidney health is a vital component of overall well-being, and what we eat plays a pivotal role in maintaining healthy kidneys. Understanding kidney-friendly diets is crucial, especially if you or a loved one is dealing with kidney-related concerns.

Kidney-friendly diets are specifically designed to support kidney function and minimize the risk of further damage. They are characterized by controlling the intake of certain nutrients such as sodium, phosphorus, and potassium, which can be problematic for those with kidney issues. These diets also focus on adequate hydration to ensure proper kidney function.

The vegan approach, which excludes animal products, can be a beneficial choice for kidney health. Let's explore the advantages of adopting a vegan kidney-friendly diet:

1. **Lower Sodium Intake**: Animal products, particularly processed meats and dairy, tend to be

high in sodium. Excess sodium can elevate blood pressure and strain the kidneys. A vegan diet naturally reduces sodium consumption, promoting better kidney health.

2. **Reduced Phosphorus**: Kidneys regulate phosphorus in the body, and high phosphorus levels can be detrimental to kidney function. Plant-based foods typically have lower levels of phosphorus, making a vegan diet kidney-friendly.

3. **Balanced Protein:** Plant-based protein sources like beans, lentils, and tofu provide a balanced protein intake without overburdening the kidneys. This is especially important for individuals with kidney issues who need to manage their protein intake.

4. **Less Potassium**: High potassium levels can be problematic for kidney patients. Vegan diets often have lower potassium content compared to animal-based diets, helping to keep potassium in check.

5. **Heart Health:** Vegan diets are associated with a reduced risk of heart disease, which is beneficial for individuals with kidney problems, as heart health and kidney health are closely intertwined.

6. **Increased Antioxidants:** Fruits and vegetables, staples of a vegan diet, are rich in antioxidants. Antioxidants help protect the kidneys from oxidative stress, promoting their longevity.

By understanding the principles of kidney-friendly diets and embracing a vegan approach, individuals can take proactive steps to support kidney health and overall well-being. It's a choice that not only benefits the kidneys but also contributes to a more sustainable and eco-friendly lifestyle.

Chapter 1: 30-Day Meal Plan

Week 1

Day 1:

- Breakfast: Creamy Oatmeal with Berries
- Lunch: Kidney Bean and Quinoa Salad
- Dinner: Vegan Eggplant Parmesan
- Snacks: Vegan Guacamole
- Dessert: Vegan Banana Ice Cream

Day 2:

- Breakfast: Vegan Scrambled Tofu
- Lunch: Vegan Lentil Soup
- Dinner: Kidney Bean Stew
- Snacks: Vegan Stuffed Mushrooms
- Dessert: Vegan Chocolate Avocado Mousse

Day 3:

- Breakfast: Sweet Potato and Spinach Breakfast Burrito
- Lunch: Spaghetti with Vegan Bolognese

- Dinner: Vegan Tofu Stir-Fry
- Snacks: Vegan Cucumber Rolls
- Dessert: Vegan Berry Parfait

Day 4:

- Breakfast: Blueberry Banana Pancakes
- Lunch: Black Bean and Corn Salad
- Dinner: Vegan Spaghetti Aglio e Olio
- Snacks: Vegan Sweet Potato Fries
- Dessert: Vegan Baked Apples

Day 5:

- Breakfast: Chia Seed Pudding
- Lunch: Vegan Falafel Wraps
- Dinner: Vegan Sweet Potato and Black Bean Chili
- Snacks: Vegan Salsa and Tortilla Chips
- Dessert: Vegan Coconut Rice Pudding

Day 6:

- Breakfast: Avocado Toast with Tomato Salsa
- Lunch: Sweet Potato and Kale Salad
- Dinner: Vegan Mushroom Risotto

* Snacks: Vegan Edamame

* Dessert: Vegan Pumpkin Pie

Day 7:

* Breakfast: Vegan Breakfast Smoothie

* Lunch: Vegan Minestrone Soup

* Dinner: Vegan Stuffed Acorn Squash

* Snacks: Vegan Greek Salad Skewers

* Dessert: Vegan Chia Seed Chocolate Pudding

Week 2

Day 8:

* Breakfast: Quinoa and Fruit Bowl

* Lunch: Spinach and Chickpea Salad

* Dinner: Vegan Teriyaki Tempeh

* Snacks: Vegan Roasted Red Pepper Dip

* Dessert: Vegan Mixed Berry Crisp

Day 9:

* Breakfast: Nutty Granola with Almond Milk

* Lunch: Vegan Thai Peanut Noodles

* Dinner: Vegan Cauliflower Curry

- Snacks: Vegan Avocado Bruschetta
- Dessert: Vegan Chocolate Chip Cookies

Day 10:

- Breakfast: Spinach and Mushroom Breakfast Quesadilla
- Lunch: Roasted Red Pepper Hummus Wrap
- Dinner: Vegan Spinach and Artichoke Pasta
- Snacks: Vegan Spinach and Artichoke Dip
- Dessert: Vegan Rice Krispie Treats

Day 11:

- Breakfast: Zucchini and Tomato Frittata
- Lunch: Vegan Sushi Bowl
- Dinner: Vegan Ratatouille
- Snacks: Vegan Hummus and Veggie Sticks
- Dessert: Vegan Lemon Sorbet

Day 12:

- Breakfast: Cinnamon Raisin French Toast
- Lunch: Vegan Butternut Squash Soup
- Dinner: Vegan Lentil Loaf

- Snacks: Vegan Fruit Salad
- Dessert: Vegan Strawberry Shortcake

Day 13:

- Breakfast: Vegan Breakfast Tacos
- Lunch: Vegan Chickpea Curry
- Dinner: Vegan Cilantro Lime Rice with Black Beans
- Snacks: Vegan Olive Tapenade
- Dessert: Vegan Blueberry Cobbler

Day 14:

- Breakfast: Peanut Butter and Banana Toast
- Lunch: Vegan Stuffed Bell Peppers
- Dinner: Vegan Portobello Steak
- Snacks: Vegan Roasted Chickpeas
- Dessert: Vegan Chocolate Covered Strawberries

Week 3

Day 15:

- Breakfast: Kidney-Friendly Green Smoothie
- Lunch: Quinoa and Avocado Salad
- Dinner: Vegan Chickpea and Spinach Curry

- Snacks: Vegan Stuffed Grape Leaves
- Dessert: Vegan Almond and Coconut Energy Balls

Day 16:

- Breakfast: Chickpea Breakfast Hash
- Lunch: Vegan Caesar Salad
- Dinner: Vegan Quinoa Stuffed Peppers
- Snacks: Vegan Zucchini Chips
- Dessert: Vegan Mango Sorbet

Day 17:

- Breakfast: Vegan Chocolate Porridge
- Lunch: Vegan Lentil Tacos
- Dinner: Vegan Thai Green Curry
- Snacks: Vegan Mini Caprese Skewers
- Dessert: Vegan Watermelon Popsicles

Day 18:

- Breakfast: Mediterranean Breakfast Bowl
- Lunch: Vegan Portobello Mushroom Burger
- Dinner: Vegan Asparagus and Lemon Risotto
- Snacks: Vegan Mixed Nuts

- Dessert: Vegan Cinnamon Baked Pears

Day 19:

- Breakfast: Creamy Oatmeal with Berries
- Lunch: Kidney Bean and Quinoa Salad
- Dinner: Vegan Eggplant Parmesan
- Snacks: Vegan Guacamole
- Dessert: Vegan Banana Ice Cream

Day 20:

- Breakfast: Vegan Scrambled Tofu
- Lunch: Vegan Lentil Soup
- Dinner: Kidney Bean Stew
- Snacks: Vegan Stuffed Mushrooms
- Dessert: Vegan Chocolate Avocado Mousse

Week 4

Day 21:

- Breakfast: Sweet Potato and Spinach Breakfast Burrito
- Lunch: Spaghetti with Vegan Bolognese
- Dinner: Vegan Tofu Stir-Fry

- Snacks: Vegan Cucumber Rolls
- Dessert: Vegan Berry Parfait

Day 22:

- Breakfast: Blueberry Banana Pancakes
- Lunch: Black Bean and Corn Salad
- Dinner: Vegan Spaghetti Aglio e Olio
- Snacks: Vegan Sweet Potato Fries
- Dessert: Vegan Baked Apples

Day 23:

- Breakfast: Chia Seed Pudding
- Lunch: Vegan Falafel Wraps
- Dinner: Vegan Sweet Potato and Black Bean Chili
- Snacks: Vegan Salsa and Tortilla Chips
- Dessert: Vegan Coconut Rice Pudding

Day 24:

- Breakfast: Avocado Toast with Tomato Salsa
- Lunch: Sweet Potato and Kale Salad
- Dinner: Vegan Mushroom Risotto
- Snacks: Vegan Edamame

- Dessert: Vegan Pumpkin Pie

Day 25:

- Breakfast: Vegan Breakfast Smoothie
- Lunch: Vegan Minestrone Soup
- Dinner: Vegan Stuffed Acorn Squash
- Snacks: Vegan Greek Salad Skewers
- Dessert: Vegan Chia Seed Chocolate Pudding

Day 26:

- Breakfast: Nutty Granola with Almond Milk
- Lunch: Vegan Thai Peanut Noodles
- Dinner: Vegan Cauliflower Curry
- Snacks: Vegan Avocado Bruschetta
- Dessert: Vegan Chocolate Chip Cookies

Day 27:

- Breakfast: Spinach and Mushroom Breakfast Quesadilla
- Lunch: Roasted Red Pepper Hummus Wrap
- Dinner: Vegan Spinach and Artichoke Pasta
- Snacks: Vegan Spinach and Artichoke Dip

- Dessert: Vegan Rice Krispie Treats

Day 28:

- Breakfast: Zucchini and Tomato Frittata
- Lunch: Vegan Sushi Bowl
- Dinner: Vegan Ratatouille
- Snacks: Vegan Hummus and Veggie Sticks
- Dessert: Vegan Lemon Sorbet

Day 29:

- Breakfast: Cinnamon Raisin French Toast
- Lunch: Vegan Butternut Squash Soup
- Dinner: Vegan Lentil Loaf
- Snacks: Vegan Fruit Salad
- Dessert: Vegan Strawberry Shortcake

Day 30:

- Breakfast: Vegan Breakfast Tacos
- Lunch: Vegan Chickpea Curry
- Dinner: Vegan Cilantro Lime Rice with Black Beans
- Snacks: Vegan Olive Tapenade
- Dessert: Vegan Blueberry Cobbler

Congratulations on completing your 30-day journey of kidney-friendly vegan meals. Enjoy the delicious and nutritious recipes!

Chapter 2: Breakfast Recipes

These recipes are not only vegan but also kidney-friendly, ensuring that you start your day with both flavor and care for your health. Whether you're a fan of the classics or prefer to explore more creative breakfast options, you'll find something here to tantalize your taste buds and nourish your body.

Creamy Oatmeal with Berries

Ingredients:

- 1 cup rolled oats
- 2 cups almond milk
- 1/2 cup mixed berries
- 1 tablespoon maple syrup
- 1/4 teaspoon cinnamon

Instructions:

1. In a saucepan, combine oats and almond milk.
2. Cook over medium heat until the oats are creamy.

3. Top with mixed berries, a drizzle of maple syrup, and
   a sprinkle of cinnamon.

Vegan Scrambled Tofu

Ingredients:

- 1/2 block firm tofu, crumbled
- 1/4 cup diced bell peppers
- 1/4 cup diced onions
- 1/4 cup spinach
- 1/2 teaspoon turmeric
- Salt and pepper to taste

Instructions:

1. Sauté bell peppers and onions until soft.
2. Add crumbled tofu, turmeric, spinach, salt, and pepper.
3. Cook until tofu is lightly browned and well-seasoned.

Sweet Potato and Spinach Breakfast Burrito

Ingredients:

- 1 large sweet potato, diced
- 1 cup fresh spinach
- 2 tortillas
- 1/4 cup black beans
- Salsa for topping

Instructions:

1. Roast sweet potato until tender.
2. Layer sweet potato, fresh spinach, and black beans on a tortilla.
3. Roll up and serve with salsa.

Blueberry Banana Pancakes

Ingredients:

- 1 cup whole wheat flour
- 1 ripe banana, mashed
- 1/2 cup blueberries
- 1 cup almond milk

- 1 tablespoon maple syrup

Instructions:

1. Mix flour, mashed banana, blueberries, almond milk, and maple syrup.
2. Cook pancakes until golden brown.

Chia Seed Pudding

Ingredients:

- 1/4 cup chia seeds
- 1 cup almond milk
- 1 tablespoon maple syrup
- 1/2 teaspoon vanilla extract
- Fresh fruit for topping

Instructions:

1. Combine chia seeds, almond milk, maple syrup, and vanilla extract.
2. Stir well and refrigerate overnight.
3. Top with fresh fruit before serving.

Avocado Toast with Tomato Salsa

Ingredients:

- 2 slices whole-grain bread
- 1 ripe avocado, mashed
- 1/2 cup diced tomatoes
- 1/4 cup red onion, finely chopped
- A pinch of salt and pepper

Instructions:

1. Spread mashed avocado on toasted bread.
2. Combine diced tomatoes and red onion with salt and pepper to make salsa.
3. Top avocado toast with the salsa.

Vegan Breakfast Smoothie

Ingredients:

- 1 ripe banana
- 1/2 cup mixed berries
- 1 cup almond milk
- 1 tablespoon chia seeds
- 1 teaspoon honey (or maple syrup for a vegan option)

Instructions:

1. Blend banana, mixed berries, almond milk, chia seeds, and honey until smooth.

Quinoa and Fruit Bowl

Ingredients:

*   1 cup cooked quinoa
*   1/2 cup mixed fresh fruit (e.g., strawberries, kiwi, and mango)
*   2 tablespoons coconut yogurt
*   1 tablespoon honey (or maple syrup)

Instructions:

1. Place cooked quinoa in a bowl.
2. Top with mixed fresh fruit, coconut yogurt, and a drizzle of honey.

Nutty Granola with Almond Milk

Ingredients:

*   1 cup vegan granola
*   1/2 cup mixed nuts (e.g., almonds and walnuts)

- Almond milk for pouring

Instructions:

1. Combine vegan granola and mixed nuts in a bowl.
2. Pour almond milk over the mixture.

Spinach and Mushroom Breakfast Quesadilla

Ingredients:

- 2 whole-grain tortillas
- 1 cup fresh spinach
- 1/2 cup sliced mushrooms
- 1/4 cup vegan cheese

Instructions:

1. Layer spinach, mushrooms, and vegan cheese between tortillas.
2. Cook until cheese is melted and tortillas are crispy.

Zucchini and Tomato Frittata

Ingredients:

- 2 cups grated zucchini
- 1 cup diced tomatoes
- 1/4 cup diced onions
- 1/4 cup chickpea flour
- 1/2 teaspoon garlic powder
- Salt and pepper to taste

Instructions:

1. Combine zucchini, tomatoes, onions, chickpea flour, garlic powder, salt, and pepper.
2. Cook in a non-stick pan until set and lightly browned.

Cinnamon Raisin French Toast

Ingredients:

- 4 slices of whole-grain bread
- 1 cup almond milk
- 1 teaspoon cinnamon
- 1/4 cup raisins
- 1 tablespoon maple syrup

Instructions:

1. Mix almond milk, cinnamon, and maple syrup.
2. Soak bread slices in the mixture and cook until golden brown.
3. Top with raisins and extra syrup.

Vegan Breakfast Tacos

Ingredients:

- 2 small whole-grain tortillas
- 1/2 cup black beans
- 1/2 cup diced avocado
- 1/4 cup salsa
- Fresh cilantro for garnish

Instructions:

1. Fill tortillas with black beans, diced avocado, and salsa.
2. Garnish with fresh cilantro.

Peanut Butter and Banana Toast

Ingredients:

- 2 slices whole-grain bread
- 2 tablespoons peanut butter
- 1 banana, sliced
- A drizzle of honey (or maple syrup)

Instructions:

1. Spread peanut butter on toasted bread.
2. Top with banana slices and a drizzle of honey.

Kidney-Friendly Green Smoothie

Ingredients:

- 1 cup fresh spinach
- 1/2 cup frozen pineapple
- 1/2 cup frozen mango
- 1/2 cup almond milk
- 1 tablespoon flaxseeds

Instructions:

1. Blend fresh spinach, frozen pineapple, frozen mango, almond milk, and flaxseeds until smooth.

Chickpea Breakfast Hash

Ingredients:

- 1 can of chickpeas, drained and rinsed
- 1 cup diced bell peppers
- 1/2 cup diced onions
- 1 teaspoon smoked paprika
- Salt and pepper to taste

Instructions:

1. Sauté chickpeas, bell peppers, and onions with smoked paprika, salt, and pepper.
2. Cook until chickpeas are slightly crispy.

Vegan Chocolate Porridge

Ingredients:

- 1 cup rolled oats
- 2 cups almond milk

- 2 tablespoons cocoa powder
- 2 tablespoons maple syrup
- Vegan chocolate chips for topping

Instructions:

1. Combine oats, almond milk, cocoa powder, and maple syrup.
2. Cook until creamy and top with vegan chocolate chips.

Mediterranean Breakfast Bowl

Ingredients:

- 1 cup cooked quinoa
- 1/2 cup cherry tomatoes, halved
- 1/4 cup diced cucumber
- 1/4 cup Kalamata olives, pitted
- 2 tablespoons hummus

Instructions:

1. Place cooked quinoa in a bowl.
2. Top with cherry tomatoes, cucumber, Kalamata olives, and a dollop of hummus.

Chapter 3: Lunch Recipes

Lunchtime offers a delightful opportunity to recharge with nourishing, kidney-friendly vegan meals. In this chapter, you'll find a diverse selection of lunch recipes that cater to your taste buds and dietary needs. Whether you're looking for a quick wrap, a hearty salad, or a comforting soup, we've got you covered.

Kidney Bean and Quinoa Salad

Ingredients:

- 1 cup cooked quinoa
- 1 can kidney beans, drained and rinsed
- 1 red bell pepper, diced
- 1/2 cucumber, diced
- 1/4 cup red onion, finely chopped
- 2 tablespoons fresh parsley, chopped
- 3 tablespoons olive oil
- 2 tablespoons red wine vinegar
- Salt and pepper to taste

Instructions:

1. In a large bowl, combine cooked quinoa, kidney beans, red bell pepper, cucumber, red onion, and parsley.
2. In a separate bowl, whisk together olive oil and red wine vinegar.
3. Pour the dressing over the salad and toss to coat.
4. Season with salt and pepper to taste.
5. Chill in the refrigerator for at least 30 minutes before serving.

Vegan Lentil Soup

Ingredients:

- 1 cup green or brown lentils, rinsed and drained
- 1 onion, chopped
- 2 carrots, chopped
- 2 celery stalks, chopped
- 3 cloves garlic, minced
- 6 cups vegetable broth
- 1 teaspoon cumin
- 1/2 teaspoon paprika
- Salt and pepper to taste

Instructions:

1. In a large pot, sauté the onion, carrots, and celery until they begin to soften.
2. Add the minced garlic and cook for an additional minute.
3. Stir in the lentils, vegetable broth, cumin, paprika, salt, and pepper.
4. Bring to a boil, then reduce the heat and let it simmer for about 30-35 minutes until the lentils are tender.
5. Blend a portion of the soup if you prefer a thicker consistency.
6. Adjust the seasoning as needed and serve hot.

Spaghetti with Vegan Bolognese

Ingredients:

- 8 oz whole wheat spaghetti
- 1 cup textured vegetable protein (TVP)
- 1 can crushed tomatoes
- 1 onion, diced
- 2 cloves garlic, minced
- 1 carrot, grated
- 1 celery stalk, chopped

- 1 teaspoon dried basil
- 1 teaspoon dried oregano
- Salt and pepper to taste

Instructions:

1. Cook spaghetti according to package instructions.
2. In a large skillet, sauté the onion, garlic, carrot, and celery until softened.
3. Add the TVP, crushed tomatoes, basil, oregano, salt, and pepper. Simmer for about 10 minutes.
4. Serve the bolognese sauce over the cooked spaghetti.

Black Bean and Corn Salad

Ingredients:

- 2 cups black beans, cooked and drained
- 1 cup corn kernels (fresh or frozen)
- 1 red bell pepper, diced
- 1/2 red onion, finely chopped
- 1/4 cup fresh cilantro, chopped
- 2 tablespoons lime juice
- 2 tablespoons olive oil
- Salt and pepper to taste

Instructions:

1. In a large bowl, combine black beans, corn, red bell pepper, red onion, and cilantro.
2. In a separate bowl, whisk together lime juice and olive oil.
3. Pour the dressing over the salad and toss to coat.
4. Season with salt and pepper to taste.
5. Chill in the refrigerator for at least 30 minutes before serving.

Vegan Falafel Wraps

Ingredients:

- 1 can chickpeas, drained and rinsed
- 2 cloves garlic, minced
- 1/4 cup fresh parsley, chopped
- 1 teaspoon ground cumin
- 1 teaspoon ground coriander
- Salt and pepper to taste
- 1/2 cup breadcrumbs
- 4 whole-wheat tortillas
- Fresh vegetables and tahini sauce for serving

Instructions:

1. In a food processor, combine chickpeas, garlic, parsley, cumin, coriander, salt, and pepper.
2. Pulse until well combined but still slightly chunky.
3. Stir in the breadcrumbs to help bind the mixture.
4. Form the mixture into small patties and fry or bake until golden brown and crispy.
5. Serve the falafel wrapped in tortillas with fresh vegetables and drizzle with tahini sauce.

Sweet Potato and Kale Salad

Ingredients:

- 2 sweet potatoes, peeled and diced
- 1 bunch kale, destemmed and chopped
- 1/4 cup dried cranberries
- 1/4 cup walnuts, chopped
- 2 tablespoons olive oil
- 1 tablespoon balsamic vinegar
- Salt and pepper to taste

Instructions:

1. Toss the sweet potatoes in olive oil and roast in the oven until tender and slightly crispy.

2. In a large bowl, massage the kale with balsamic vinegar until it softens.

3. Combine roasted sweet potatoes, kale, dried cranberries, and chopped walnuts.

4. Season with salt and pepper, and serve as a nutritious salad.

Vegan Minestrone Soup

Ingredients:

- 1 cup small pasta (such as ditalini)
- 1 can kidney beans, drained and rinsed
- 1 zucchini, diced
- 1 carrot, diced
- 1 celery stalk, diced
- 1 can diced tomatoes
- 1 onion, chopped
- 2 cloves garlic, minced
- 6 cups vegetable broth
- 1 teaspoon dried basil

- 1 teaspoon dried oregano
- Salt and pepper to taste

Instructions:

1. Cook the pasta separately according to the package instructions.
2. In a large pot, sauté the onion, garlic, carrot, and celery until softened.
3. Add the zucchini, kidney beans, diced tomatoes, vegetable broth, basil, oregano, salt, and pepper.
4. Simmer for about 15 minutes until the vegetables are tender.
5. Serve the minestrone soup with cooked pasta.

Spinach and Chickpea Salad

Ingredients:

- 4 cups fresh spinach leaves
- 1 can chickpeas, drained and rinsed
- 1/4 red onion, finely chopped
- 1/4 cup cherry tomatoes, halved
- 2 tablespoons balsamic vinaigrette
- Salt and pepper to taste

Instructions:

1. In a large bowl, combine fresh spinach, chickpeas, red onion, and cherry tomatoes.

2. Drizzle with balsamic vinaigrette and toss to coat.

3. Season with salt and pepper as desired.

Vegan Thai Peanut Noodles

Ingredients:

- 8 oz rice noodles
- 1/4 cup peanut butter
- 2 tablespoons soy sauce
- 1 tablespoon lime juice
- 1 tablespoon maple syrup
- 1/2 teaspoon sriracha sauce (adjust to taste)
- 1 cup broccoli florets, steamed
- 1 carrot, julienned
- 1/4 cup peanuts, chopped
- Fresh cilantro for garnish

Instructions:

1. Cook rice noodles according to package instructions and set aside.

2. In a bowl, whisk together peanut butter, soy sauce, lime juice, maple syrup, and sriracha sauce until smooth.

3. Toss the cooked noodles with the peanut sauce, steamed broccoli, and julienned carrots.

4. Garnish with chopped peanuts and fresh cilantro.

Roasted Red Pepper Hummus Wrap

Ingredients:

- 1 whole-wheat wrap
- 1/2 cup roasted red pepper hummus
- 1 cup mixed greens
- 1/2 cucumber, thinly sliced
- 1/4 red onion, thinly sliced
- Salt and pepper to taste

Instructions:

1. Spread roasted red pepper hummus evenly on the whole-wheat wrap.

2. Layer on mixed greens, cucumber slices, and red onion.

3. Season with salt and pepper.

4. Roll the wrap tightly and enjoy!

Vegan Sushi Bowl

Ingredients:

- 2 cups cooked sushi rice
- 1 avocado, sliced
- 1/2 cucumber, diced
- 1 carrot, julienned
- 1/2 nori sheet, shredded
- Soy sauce or tamari for drizzling
- Pickled ginger and wasabi for serving

Instructions:

1. In a bowl, arrange sushi rice and top with avocado, cucumber, carrot, and shredded nori.
2. Drizzle with soy sauce or tamari to taste.
3. Serve with pickled ginger and wasabi on the side.

Vegan Butternut Squash Soup

Ingredients:

- 1 butternut squash, peeled, seeded, and cubed

- 1 onion, chopped
- 2 carrots, chopped
- 2 apples, peeled, cored, and chopped
- 4 cups vegetable broth
- 1 teaspoon cinnamon
- 1/2 teaspoon nutmeg
- Salt and pepper to taste

Instructions:

1. In a large pot, sauté the onion, carrots, and apples until they begin to soften.
2. Add the cubed butternut squash, vegetable broth, cinnamon, nutmeg, salt, and pepper.
3. Simmer for about 20-25 minutes until the vegetables are tender.
4. Blend the soup until smooth and adjust seasoning as needed.

Vegan Chickpea Curry

Ingredients:

- 1 can chickpeas, drained and rinsed
- 1 onion, chopped

- 2 cloves garlic, minced
- 1 can diced tomatoes
- 1 cup coconut milk
- 2 tablespoons curry powder
- Salt and pepper to taste

Instructions:

1. In a skillet, sauté the onion and garlic until softened.
2. Add chickpeas, diced tomatoes, coconut milk, curry powder, salt, and pepper.
3. Simmer for about 15 minutes, stirring occasionally.
4. Serve the chickpea curry with rice or bread.

Vegan Stuffed Bell Peppers

Ingredients:

- 4 bell peppers, tops removed and seeds removed
- 1 cup cooked quinoa
- 1 can black beans, drained and rinsed
- 1 cup corn kernels (fresh or frozen)
- 1/2 cup diced tomatoes
- 1/2 teaspoon chili powder
- 1/2 teaspoon cumin

- Salt and pepper to taste

Instructions:

1. Preheat the oven to 350°F (175°C).
2. In a bowl, mix cooked quinoa, black beans, corn, diced tomatoes, chili powder, cumin, salt, and pepper.
3. Stuff each bell pepper with the mixture.
4. Place the stuffed peppers in a baking dish and cover with foil.
5. Bake for about 30-35 minutes until the peppers are tender.

Quinoa and Avocado Salad

Ingredients:

- 1 cup cooked quinoa
- 1 avocado, diced
- 1/2 cup cherry tomatoes, halved
- 1/4 cup red onion, finely chopped
- 2 tablespoons fresh cilantro, chopped
- 2 tablespoons lime juice
- 2 tablespoons olive oil

- Salt and pepper to taste

Instructions:

1. In a bowl, combine cooked quinoa, diced avocado, cherry tomatoes, red onion, and cilantro.
2. In a separate bowl, whisk together lime juice and olive oil.
3. Pour the dressing over the salad and toss to coat.
4. Season with salt and pepper to taste.

Vegan Caesar Salad

Ingredients:

- 1 head romaine lettuce, chopped
- 1/2 cup croutons (look for low-sodium options)
- Vegan Caesar dressing (store-bought or homemade)
- Vegan parmesan cheese for garnish (optional)

Instructions:

1. In a large bowl, combine chopped romaine lettuce and croutons.
2. Drizzle with your preferred vegan Caesar dressing and toss to coat.

3. Garnish with vegan parmesan cheese if desired.

Vegan Lentil Tacos

Ingredients:

- 1 cup brown or green lentils, cooked and drained
- 1 tablespoon taco seasoning
- 1 cup lettuce, shredded
- 1/2 cup diced tomatoes
- 1/4 cup diced red onion
- 1/4 cup dairy-free yogurt (as a topping)
- Whole-wheat tortillas

Instructions:

1. In a skillet, heat cooked lentils and taco seasoning until heated through.
2. Assemble tacos by placing lentils, lettuce, tomatoes, and red onion on tortillas.
3. Top with dairy-free yogurt.

Vegan Portobello Mushroom Burger

Ingredients:

- 2 large Portobello mushroom caps
- 1/4 cup balsamic vinegar
- 2 cloves garlic, minced
- 2 whole-wheat burger buns
- Vegan burger toppings of your choice (lettuce, tomato, onion, vegan cheese, etc.)

Instructions:

1. In a bowl, mix balsamic vinegar and minced garlic.
2. Marinate Portobello mushroom caps in the mixture for about 15 minutes.
3. Grill or roast the mushrooms until tender, about 10-15 minutes.
4. Assemble the mushrooms on whole-wheat burger buns with your favorite toppings.

Chapter 4: Dinner Recipes

In this chapter, we embark on a delectable journey through an array of wholesome vegan dinner recipes, meticulously crafted to delight your taste buds while prioritizing kidney health. Each dish offers a unique combination of flavors and textures, making your evening meal an exciting and nutritious experience.

Vegan Eggplant Parmesan

Ingredients:

- 1 large eggplant, sliced
- 1 cup of breadcrumbs
- 1 cup of vegan mozzarella cheese
- 2 cups of tomato sauce
- 1 tablespoon of olive oil
- Fresh basil leaves for garnish

Instructions:

1. Preheat the oven to 375°F (190°C).

2. Dip eggplant slices in olive oil, then coat with breadcrumbs.

3. Arrange slices in a baking dish, layer with tomato sauce and vegan mozzarella.

4. Bake for 25-30 minutes until the cheese is bubbly and golden.

5. Garnish with fresh basil.

Kidney Bean Stew

Ingredients:

- 1 cup of kidney beans, soaked and cooked
- 1 onion, chopped
- 2 cloves of garlic, minced
- 2 carrots, sliced
- 1 bell pepper, diced
- 1 can of diced tomatoes
- 4 cups of vegetable broth
- 1 teaspoon of cumin
- 1 teaspoon of paprika
- Salt and pepper to taste

Instructions:

1. Sauté onions and garlic in a large pot until translucent.
2. Add carrots, bell pepper, kidney beans, and spices. Cook for a few minutes.
3. Pour in diced tomatoes and vegetable broth.
4. Simmer for 30 minutes or until the vegetables are tender.

Vegan Tofu Stir-Fry

Ingredients:

- 1 block of firm tofu, cubed
- 2 cups of mixed vegetables (broccoli, bell peppers, carrots)
- 2 cloves of garlic, minced
- 1/4 cup of soy sauce
- 1 tablespoon of sesame oil
- 1 tablespoon of cornstarch

Instructions:

1. In a bowl, mix soy sauce, sesame oil, and cornstarch.
2. Stir-fry tofu in a pan until golden, then remove.

3. In the same pan, stir-fry garlic and vegetables.

4. Add the sauce and tofu. Cook until heated through.

Vegan Spaghetti Aglio e Olio

Ingredients:

- 8 oz of whole wheat spaghetti
- 4 cloves of garlic, thinly sliced
- 1/4 cup of olive oil
- Red pepper flakes (to taste)
- Fresh parsley, chopped
- Salt and black pepper

Instructions:

1. Cook spaghetti according to package instructions.
2. In a pan, sauté garlic in olive oil until golden.
3. Add red pepper flakes, salt, and black pepper.
4. Toss cooked pasta in the garlic oil.
5. Garnish with fresh parsley.

Vegan Sweet Potato and Black Bean Chili

Ingredients:

- 2 large sweet potatoes, diced
- 1 can of black beans, drained and rinsed
- 1 onion, chopped
- 2 cloves of garlic, minced
- 1 can of diced tomatoes
- 2 cups of vegetable broth
- 2 tablespoons of chili powder
- 1 teaspoon of cumin
- Salt and pepper to taste

Instructions:

1. In a large pot, sauté onions and garlic until fragrant.
2. Add sweet potatoes, black beans, diced tomatoes, and spices.
3. Pour in vegetable broth and simmer for 25-30 minutes.

Vegan Mushroom Risotto

Ingredients:

- 1 1/2 cups of Arborio rice
- 1 lb of mushrooms, sliced
- 1 onion, chopped
- 4 cups of vegetable broth
- 1/2 cup of white wine (optional)
- 2 tablespoons of olive oil
- 2 cloves of garlic, minced
- 1/4 cup of vegan Parmesan cheese
- Salt and pepper to taste

Instructions:

1. In a large skillet, sauté onions, garlic, and mushrooms in olive oil.
2. Stir in Arborio rice and cook for a few minutes.
3. Add white wine (if using) and allow it to evaporate.
4. Gradually add vegetable broth, stirring until absorbed.
5. Stir in vegan Parmesan cheese, salt, and pepper.

Vegan Stuffed Acorn Squash

Ingredients:

- 2 acorn squash, halved and seeds removed
- 1 cup of quinoa
- 2 cups of vegetable broth
- 1 onion, chopped
- 2 cloves of garlic, minced
- 1/2 cup of dried cranberries
- 1/2 cup of chopped pecans
- 1/4 cup of fresh parsley, chopped
- 2 tablespoons of olive oil
- Salt and pepper to taste

Instructions:

1. Preheat the oven to 375°F (190°C).
2. Place acorn squash halves on a baking sheet, brush with olive oil, and roast for 30-40 minutes.
3. In a saucepan, sauté onions and garlic, then add quinoa and vegetable broth. Cook until fluffy.
4. Stir in cranberries, pecans, parsley, salt, and pepper.
5. Stuff the roasted acorn squash with the quinoa mixture.

Vegan Teriyaki Tempeh

Ingredients:

- 1 package of tempeh, cubed
- 1/4 cup of teriyaki sauce
- 2 tablespoons of sesame oil
- 2 cloves of garlic, minced
- 1 tablespoon of sesame seeds
- Sliced green onions for garnish

Instructions:

1. In a pan, sauté tempeh in sesame oil until browned.
2. Add minced garlic and teriyaki sauce.
3. Simmer until the sauce thickens.
4. Sprinkle with sesame seeds and garnish with sliced green onions.

Vegan Cauliflower Curry

Ingredients:

- 1 small cauliflower, cut into florets
- 1 can of chickpeas, drained and rinsed
- 1 onion, chopped

- 2 cloves of garlic, minced
- 1 can of diced tomatoes
- 1 can of coconut milk
- 2 tablespoons of curry powder
- Salt and pepper to taste
- Fresh cilantro for garnish

Instructions:

1. In a pot, sauté onions and garlic until softened.
2. Add cauliflower, chickpeas, diced tomatoes, coconut milk, and curry powder.
3. Simmer until cauliflower is tender.
4. Season with salt and pepper, garnish with fresh cilantro.

Vegan Spinach and Artichoke Pasta

Ingredients:

- 8 oz of whole wheat pasta
- 2 cups of fresh spinach
- 1 can of artichoke hearts, chopped
- 1 onion, chopped
- 2 cloves of garlic, minced

- 1/4 cup of vegan cream cheese
- 1/4 cup of nutritional yeast
- Salt and black pepper to taste

Instructions:

1. Cook pasta according to package instructions.
2. In a pan, sauté onions and garlic until translucent.
3. Add spinach and chopped artichoke hearts.
4. Stir in vegan cream cheese and nutritional yeast.
5. Toss cooked pasta in the creamy spinach mixture.

Vegan Ratatouille

Ingredients:

- 1 eggplant, sliced
- 2 zucchinis, sliced
- 2 tomatoes, sliced
- 1 onion, sliced
- 2 cloves of garlic, minced
- 2 tablespoons of olive oil
- Fresh thyme and rosemary
- Salt and pepper to taste

Instructions:

1. Preheat the oven to 375°F (190°C).
2. In a baking dish, layer eggplant, zucchinis, tomatoes, and onions.
3. Drizzle with olive oil and sprinkle garlic, thyme, rosemary, salt, and pepper.
4. Bake for 40-45 minutes until the vegetables are tender.

Vegan Lentil Loaf

Ingredients:

- 1 cup of green or brown lentils, cooked
- 1 onion, chopped
- 2 cloves of garlic, minced
- 1 carrot, grated
- 1/2 cup of oats
- 1/2 cup of breadcrumbs
- 1/4 cup of ketchup
- 2 tablespoons of soy sauce
- 1 teaspoon of dried thyme
- Salt and pepper to taste

Instructions:

1. Preheat the oven to 350°F (175°C).

2. Sauté onions and garlic until softened.

3. In a bowl, combine lentils, grated carrot, oats, breadcrumbs, ketchup, soy sauce, thyme, salt, and pepper.

4. Transfer the mixture to a loaf pan.

5. Bake for 45-50 minutes until the loaf is firm.

Vegan Cilantro Lime Rice with Black Beans

Ingredients:

- 1 cup of white rice
- 1 can of black beans, drained and rinsed
- Zest and juice of 2 limes
- 1/4 cup of fresh cilantro, chopped
- 2 cloves of garlic, minced
- Salt and black pepper to taste

Instructions:

1. Cook rice according to package instructions.

2. In a bowl, combine cooked rice, black beans, lime zest, lime juice, cilantro, and minced garlic.

3. Season with salt and black pepper.

Vegan Portobello Steak

Ingredients:

- 4 large Portobello mushrooms
- 1/4 cup of balsamic vinegar
- 2 tablespoons of olive oil
- 2 cloves of garlic, minced
- 1 teaspoon of dried rosemary
- Salt and black pepper to taste

Instructions:

1. In a bowl, whisk together balsamic vinegar, olive oil, garlic, rosemary, salt, and black pepper.

2. Brush the mixture over Portobello mushrooms.

3. Grill or bake mushrooms until tender, basting with the marinade.

Vegan Chickpea and Spinach Curry

Ingredients:

- 1 can of chickpeas, drained and rinsed
- 4 cups of fresh spinach
- 1 onion, chopped
- 2 cloves of garlic, minced
- 1 can of coconut milk
- 2 tablespoons of curry powder
- Salt and pepper to taste

Instructions:

1. Sauté onions and garlic until softened.
2. Add chickpeas, fresh spinach, coconut milk, and curry powder.
3. Simmer until the spinach wilts.
4. Season with salt and pepper.

Vegan Quinoa Stuffed Peppers

Ingredients:

- 4 large bell peppers
- 1 cup of quinoa, cooked

- 1 can of black beans, drained and rinsed
- 1 cup of corn kernels
- 1 cup of diced tomatoes
- 1 teaspoon of chili powder
- Salt and pepper to taste

Instructions:

1. Preheat the oven to 350°F (175°C).
2. Cut the tops off bell peppers and remove seeds.
3. In a bowl, mix cooked quinoa, black beans, corn, diced tomatoes, chili powder, salt, and pepper.
4. Stuff the peppers with the quinoa mixture.
5. Bake for 25-30 minutes until peppers are tender.

Vegan Thai Green Curry

Ingredients:

- 1 can of coconut milk
- 2 tablespoons of green curry paste
- 1 cup of broccoli florets
- 1 bell pepper, sliced
- 1 cup of sliced carrots
- 1 cup of sliced zucchini

- 1 block of firm tofu, cubed
- Fresh basil leaves for garnish
- Cooked rice for serving

Instructions:

1. In a large pan, simmer coconut milk and green curry paste.
2. Add broccoli, bell pepper, carrots, and zucchini.
3. Stir in cubed tofu and cook until vegetables are tender.
4. Serve over cooked rice and garnish with fresh basil.

Vegan Asparagus and Lemon Risotto

Ingredients:

- 1 1/2 cups of Arborio rice
- 1 lb of asparagus, trimmed and cut into pieces
- 1 onion, chopped
- 2 cloves of garlic, minced
- Zest and juice of 1 lemon
- 4 cups of vegetable broth

- 2 tablespoons of olive oil
- Salt and black pepper to taste

Instructions:

1. In a large skillet, sauté onions and garlic in olive oil.
2. Add Arborio rice and cook for a few minutes.
3. Gradually add vegetable broth, stirring until absorbed.
4. Stir in asparagus, lemon zest, and lemon juice.
5. Cook until rice is creamy and asparagus is tender.

Chapter 5: Snacks and Appetizers

In this section, we dive into a delightful array of vegan snacks and appetizers that will satisfy your cravings and impress your guests. These recipes are not only delicious but also kind to your kidneys. Let's explore a world of flavors and textures that make for perfect starters or midday munchies.

Vegan Guacamole

Ingredients:

- 2 ripe avocados
- 1 small red onion, finely diced
- 1-2 cloves garlic, minced
- 1-2 ripe tomatoes, diced
- 1 lime, juiced
- Salt and pepper to taste
- Fresh cilantro, chopped (for garnish)

Instructions:

1. Cut the avocados in half, remove the pit, and scoop out the flesh.
2. Mash the avocados in a bowl.
3. Add the diced onion, minced garlic, and diced tomatoes to the mashed avocados.
4. Squeeze the lime juice over the mixture and season with salt and pepper.
5. Mix everything together and garnish with fresh cilantro.
6. Serve with tortilla chips or veggie sticks.

Vegan Stuffed Mushrooms

Ingredients:

- 12 large mushroom caps
- 1/2 cup vegan cream cheese
- 2 cloves garlic, minced
- 1/4 cup breadcrumbs
- Fresh parsley, chopped (for garnish)

Instructions:

1. Preheat your oven to 375°F (190°C).

2. Remove the stems from the mushroom caps and set them aside.

3. In a bowl, mix the vegan cream cheese, minced garlic, and breadcrumbs.

4. Stuff each mushroom cap with the cream cheese mixture.

5. Place the stuffed mushrooms on a baking sheet.

6. Bake for 15-20 minutes or until they're golden and bubbling.

7. Garnish with chopped fresh parsley before serving.

Vegan Cucumber Rolls

Ingredients:

- 2 large cucumbers
- 1 cup hummus
- 1 red bell pepper, thinly sliced
- 1 carrot, julienned
- Fresh dill (for garnish)

Instructions:

1. Slice the cucumbers lengthwise into thin strips using a peeler.

2. Spread a layer of hummus onto each cucumber strip.

3. Place a few slices of red bell pepper and julienned carrot on top of the hummus.

4. Roll up the cucumber strips and secure with toothpicks.

5. Garnish with fresh dill and serve.

Vegan Sweet Potato Fries

Ingredients:

- 2 large sweet potatoes
- 2 tablespoons olive oil
- 1 teaspoon paprika
- 1/2 teaspoon salt
- 1/4 teaspoon black pepper

Instructions:

1. Preheat your oven to 425°F (220°C).

2. Peel the sweet potatoes and cut them into thin fries.

3. In a large bowl, toss the sweet potato fries with olive oil, paprika, salt, and pepper.

4. Spread the fries in a single layer on a baking sheet.

5. Bake for 20-25 minutes or until they're crispy and golden.

Vegan Salsa and Tortilla Chips

Ingredients for Salsa:

- 3 ripe tomatoes, diced
- 1 red onion, finely chopped
- 1/4 cup fresh cilantro, chopped
- 1-2 jalapeño peppers, finely chopped
- 1 lime, juiced
- Salt and pepper to taste

Ingredients for Tortilla Chips:

- Corn tortillas
- Olive oil
- Salt

Instructions for Salsa:

1. In a bowl, combine the diced tomatoes, chopped red onion, cilantro, and jalapeño peppers.
2. Squeeze the lime juice over the mixture and season with salt and pepper.

3. Mix well and let it sit for a while for the flavors to meld.

Instructions for Tortilla Chips:
1. Preheat your oven to 350°F (175°C).
2. Cut the corn tortillas into triangles.
3. Brush them lightly with olive oil and sprinkle with salt.
4. Arrange the tortilla triangles on a baking sheet.
5. Bake for 10-12 minutes or until they're crispy.

Vegan Edamame

Ingredients:
- 1 cup edamame pods (frozen or fresh)
- Salt to taste

Instructions:
1. Boil a pot of water and add a pinch of salt.
2. Add the edamame pods and boil for 3-5 minutes (or 1-2 minutes for frozen edamame).
3. Drain and serve with an extra sprinkle of salt.

Vegan Greek Salad Skewers

Ingredients:

- Cherry tomatoes
- Cucumber, cut into chunks
- Kalamata olives
- Vegan feta cheese, cubed
- Fresh oregano leaves
- Balsamic glaze (optional)

Instructions:

1. Assemble the cherry tomatoes, cucumber, Kalamata olives, vegan feta cheese, and fresh oregano leaves onto skewers.
2. Drizzle with balsamic glaze if desired.

Vegan Roasted Red Pepper Dip

Ingredients:

- 2 red bell peppers
- 1 cup raw cashews, soaked
- 2 cloves garlic, minced
- 2 tablespoons lemon juice

* 2 tablespoons nutritional yeast
* Salt and pepper to taste

Instructions:

1. Roast the red bell peppers until the skin is charred, then peel and deseed them.
2. In a blender, combine the roasted red peppers, soaked cashews, minced garlic, lemon juice, nutritional yeast, salt, and pepper.
3. Blend until smooth and creamy.
4. Serve as a dip with fresh veggies or pita bread.

Vegan Avocado Bruschetta

Ingredients:

* Baguette slices
* 2 ripe avocados
* 1 clove garlic, minced
* Cherry tomatoes, diced
* Fresh basil leaves, chopped
* Balsamic glaze (optional)

Instructions:

1. Toast the baguette slices.

2. Mash the ripe avocados and mix with minced garlic.

3. Top the toasted baguette with the avocado mixture, diced cherry tomatoes, and fresh basil.

4. Drizzle with balsamic glaze if desired.

Vegan Spinach and Artichoke Dip

Ingredients:

-   1 cup frozen chopped spinach, thawed and drained
-   1 can (14 oz) artichoke hearts, drained and chopped
-   1 cup vegan mayonnaise
-   1 cup vegan cream cheese
-   1/2 cup nutritional yeast
-   1 teaspoon garlic powder
-   Salt and pepper to taste

Instructions:

1. Preheat your oven to 375°F (190°C).

2. In a mixing bowl, combine the chopped spinach, chopped artichoke hearts, vegan mayonnaise, vegan cream cheese, nutritional yeast, and garlic powder.

3. Season with salt and pepper.

4. Transfer the mixture to a baking dish.

5. Bake for 25-30 minutes or until it's hot and bubbly.

6. Serve with tortilla chips, veggie sticks, or crackers.

Vegan Hummus and Veggie Sticks

Ingredients:

- Your favorite store-bought or homemade hummus
- Carrot sticks
- Celery sticks
- Cucumber sticks
- Bell pepper strips

Instructions:

1. Arrange the veggie sticks on a platter alongside a bowl of hummus.

2. Dip and enjoy!

Vegan Fruit Salad

Ingredients:

- Assorted fresh fruits (e.g., strawberries, blueberries, melon, kiwi, grapes)
- Fresh mint leaves (for garnish)
- Lime or lemon juice (optional)

Instructions:

1. Wash, peel (if necessary), and chop the fresh fruits.
2. Combine them in a large bowl.
3. Drizzle with lime or lemon juice for extra flavor if desired.
4. Garnish with fresh mint leaves.

Vegan Olive Tapenade

Ingredients:

- 1 cup pitted black olives
- 1/4 cup capers
- 2 cloves garlic
- 2 tablespoons lemon juice
- 2 tablespoons olive oil

- Fresh basil leaves (for garnish)

Instructions:

1. In a food processor, combine the pitted black olives, capers, minced garlic, lemon juice, and olive oil.
2. Blend until you achieve a chunky paste.
3. Garnish with fresh basil leaves.
4. Serve with bread or crackers.

Vegan Roasted Chickpeas

Ingredients:

- 1 can (15 oz) chickpeas, drained and rinsed
- 1-2 tablespoons olive oil
- Seasonings of your choice (e.g., paprika, cumin, garlic powder, cayenne pepper)
- Salt to taste

Instructions:

1. Preheat your oven to 400°F (200°C).
2. Toss the chickpeas with olive oil and your choice of seasonings.
3. Spread them on a baking sheet.

4. Roast for 25-30 minutes or until they're crispy.

Vegan Stuffed Grape Leaves

Ingredients:

- 1 jar grape leaves
- 1 cup cooked quinoa
- 1/2 cup chopped fresh parsley
- 1/4 cup chopped fresh mint
- 1/4 cup lemon juice
- Salt and pepper to taste

Instructions:

1. Rinse and drain the grape leaves.
2. In a bowl, mix cooked quinoa, chopped parsley, chopped mint, lemon juice, salt, and pepper.
3. Place a grape leaf on a flat surface, add a spoonful of the quinoa mixture, and roll it up.
4. Serve cold or at room temperature.

Vegan Zucchini Chips

Ingredients:

- Zucchini, thinly sliced
- Olive oil
- Salt and your choice of seasonings

Instructions:

1. Preheat your oven to 225°F (110°C).
2. Toss the zucchini slices with olive oil, salt, and your preferred seasonings.
3. Arrange the slices on a baking sheet.
4. Bake for 1.5-2 hours or until they're crisp.

Vegan Mini Caprese Skewers

Ingredients:

- Cherry tomatoes
- Vegan mozzarella balls
- Fresh basil leaves
- Balsamic glaze (optional)

Instructions:

1. Assemble cherry tomatoes, vegan mozzarella balls, and fresh basil leaves onto skewers.
2. Drizzle with balsamic glaze if desired.

Vegan Mixed Nuts

Ingredients:

- A mix of your favorite raw or roasted nuts (e.g., almonds, cashews, walnuts, peanuts)
- A pinch of sea salt

Instructions:

1. Simply serve a bowl of mixed nuts with a pinch of sea salt for an easy and satisfying snack.

Chapter 6: Desserts

Indulging in delightful desserts is one of the sweetest pleasures in life, and being on a kidney-friendly vegan diet doesn't mean you have to miss out. In this chapter, we present a collection of delectable desserts that are not only delicious but also suitable for kidney health.

Vegan Banana Ice Cream

Ingredients:

- 3 ripe bananas
- 1 teaspoon vanilla extract
- 1/4 cup almond milk
- Toppings of your choice (berries, nuts, or dark chocolate chips)

Instructions:

1. Slice the ripe bananas and freeze them for at least 2 hours.
2. In a food processor, blend the frozen banana slices, vanilla extract, and almond milk until creamy.

3. Serve with your favorite toppings.

Vegan Chocolate Avocado Mousse

Ingredients:

- 2 ripe avocados
- 1/4 cup cocoa powder
- 1/4 cup maple syrup
- 1 teaspoon vanilla extract

Instructions:

1. Scoop out the flesh from the avocados and blend with cocoa powder, maple syrup, and vanilla extract until smooth.
2. Chill in the fridge for 30 minutes before serving.

Vegan Berry Parfait

Ingredients:

- 1 cup mixed berries (strawberries, blueberries, raspberries)
- 1 cup vegan yogurt
- 1/2 cup granola

- 1 tablespoon maple syrup

Instructions:

1. In a glass, layer the vegan yogurt, mixed berries, and granola.
2. Drizzle maple syrup on top.

Vegan Baked Apples

Ingredients:

- 4 apples
- 1/4 cup chopped nuts (e.g., walnuts or almonds)
- 2 tablespoons maple syrup
- 1 teaspoon ground cinnamon

Instructions:

1. Core the apples and stuff them with chopped nuts, maple syrup, and ground cinnamon.
2. Bake at 350°F (175°C) for 25-30 minutes.

Vegan Coconut Rice Pudding

Ingredients:

- 1 cup cooked rice
- 1 can (14 oz) coconut milk
- 1/4 cup maple syrup
- 1/2 teaspoon vanilla extract

Instructions:

1. In a saucepan, combine cooked rice, coconut milk, maple syrup, and vanilla extract.
2. Simmer over low heat until the mixture thickens.

Vegan Pumpkin Pie

Ingredients:

- 1 prepared vegan pie crust
- 1 can (15 oz) pumpkin puree
- 1/2 cup coconut milk
- 1/2 cup maple syrup
- 1 teaspoon pumpkin pie spice

Instructions:

1. Preheat the oven to 350°F (175°C).

2. In a bowl, combine pumpkin puree, coconut milk, maple syrup, and pumpkin pie spice.

3. Pour the mixture into the pie crust and bake for 45-50 minutes.

Vegan Chia Seed Chocolate Pudding

Ingredients:

- 1/4 cup chia seeds
- 1 cup almond milk
- 2 tablespoons cocoa powder
- 1 tablespoon maple syrup

Instructions:

1. Mix chia seeds, almond milk, cocoa powder, and maple syrup in a jar.

2. Refrigerate for at least 3 hours, stirring occasionally until it thickens.

Vegan Mixed Berry Crisp

Ingredients:

- 2 cups mixed berries
- 1/2 cup rolled oats
- 1/4 cup almond flour
- 2 tablespoons maple syrup
- 1/4 teaspoon cinnamon

Instructions:

1. In a baking dish, mix mixed berries with maple syrup.
2. In a separate bowl, combine rolled oats, almond flour, and cinnamon.
3. Sprinkle the oat mixture over the berries and bake at 350°F (175°C) for 25-30 minutes.

Vegan Chocolate Chip Cookies

Ingredients:

- 1 cup almond flour
- 1/4 cup coconut oil
- 1/4 cup maple syrup

- 1/2 cup vegan chocolate chips

Instructions:

1. Preheat the oven to 350°F (175°C).

2. Mix almond flour, melted coconut oil, and maple syrup until a dough forms.

3. Stir in the chocolate chips, then drop spoonfuls onto a baking sheet and bake for 12-15 minutes.

Vegan Rice Krispie Treats

Ingredients:

- 6 cups crispy rice cereal
- 1/4 cup coconut oil
- 1/2 cup vegan marshmallows
- 1/4 cup almond butter

Instructions:

1. In a large pot, melt coconut oil, vegan marshmallows, and almond butter.

2. Stir in the crispy rice cereal, then press the mixture into a greased pan. Let it cool before cutting.

Vegan Lemon Sorbet

Ingredients:

- 3-4 lemons, juiced and zested
- 1/2 cup sugar
- 1 cup water

Instructions:

1. Heat water and sugar in a saucepan until the sugar dissolves to make a simple syrup.
2. Stir in lemon juice and zest.
3. Freeze the mixture in an ice cream maker or a shallow container, stirring occasionally until firm.

Vegan Strawberry Shortcake

Ingredients:

- 1 cup vegan shortcake biscuits
- 1 cup sliced strawberries
- 1/2 cup vegan whipped cream

Instructions:

1. Slice the shortcake biscuits in half.

2. Layer with sliced strawberries and a dollop of vegan whipped cream.

Vegan Blueberry Cobbler

Ingredients:

- 2 cups blueberries
- 1 cup almond flour
- 1/4 cup coconut oil
- 1/4 cup maple syrup

Instructions:

1. In a baking dish, mix blueberries with maple syrup.
2. In a bowl, combine almond flour and melted coconut oil. Crumble this mixture on top of the blueberries.
3. Bake at 350°F (175°C) for 30-35 minutes.

Vegan Chocolate Covered Strawberries

Ingredients:

- Fresh strawberries
- Vegan chocolate chips

Instructions:

1. Melt vegan chocolate chips in a microwave or double boiler.

2. Dip strawberries in melted chocolate and let them cool on parchment paper.

Vegan Almond and Coconut Energy Balls

Ingredients:

- 1 cup dates, pitted
- 1/2 cup almonds
- 1/4 cup shredded coconut

Instructions:

1. Blend dates and almonds in a food processor until a sticky dough forms.

2. Roll the dough into bite-sized balls and coat with shredded coconut.

Vegan Mango Sorbet

Ingredients:

- 2 ripe mangoes, peeled and diced
- 1/4 cup lime juice
- 1/4 cup maple syrup

Instructions:

1. Blend the mangoes, lime juice, and maple syrup in a blender until smooth.
2. Freeze the mixture in an ice cream maker or a shallow container, stirring occasionally until firm.

Vegan Watermelon Popsicles

Ingredients:

- 2 cups watermelon, diced
- 1/4 cup lime juice
- 1 tablespoon agave nectar

Instructions:

1. Blend watermelon, lime juice, and agave nectar.
2. Pour into popsicle molds and freeze.

Vegan Cinnamon Baked Pears

Ingredients:

- 4 ripe pears, halved and cored
- 2 tablespoons maple syrup
- 1 teaspoon ground cinnamon

Instructions:

1. Preheat the oven to 375°F (190°C).
2. Place pear halves on a baking sheet, drizzle with maple syrup, and sprinkle with cinnamon.
3. Bake for 25-30 minutes until tender.

CONCLUSION

In the culinary journey we've embarked on throughout this cookbook, we've explored the delightful realm of kidney-friendly vegan cuisine. As we reach the final chapter, it's not just an end but a beginning. The conclusion of this book marks a stepping stone towards a healthier and more conscious way of living and eating.

In the midst of these carefully crafted recipes, you've not only discovered the tantalizing flavors of plant-based ingredients but also the nurturing impact they can have on kidney health. It's a testament to the versatility and creativity of vegan cooking, showing that you can savor mouthwatering dishes while prioritizing your well-being.

As you conclude this book, consider it a launching pad for your ongoing journey to a healthier lifestyle. Beyond these recipes, there's a whole world of plant-based, kidney-friendly options waiting to be explored. Embrace the knowledge you've gained here, and let it empower you to make informed choices about your diet.

Remember that every meal you prepare using the recipes in this cookbook is a conscious step towards a better, healthier you. Your journey towards kidney health is not a sprint but a marathon, and this cookbook is just the beginning of a long and fulfilling adventure.

We hope you've enjoyed this cookbook as much as we've enjoyed creating it. May the flavors linger in your memory, and may your journey to kidney wellness be vibrant and rewarding. Thank you for joining us on this delicious and nourishing expedition.